Mediterranean Dash Diet Cookbook 2021

An Unmissable Recipe Collection for Your Mediterranean Dash Diet Meals

Kathyrn Solano

© Copyright 2021 - All rights reserved.

The content contained within this book may not be reproduced, duplicated or transmitted without direct written permission from the author or the publisher.

Under no circumstances will any blame or legal responsibility be held against the publisher, or author, for any damages, reparation, or monetary loss due to the information contained within this book. Either directly or indirectly.

Legal Notice:

This book is copyright protected. This book is only for personal use. You cannot amend, distribute, sell, use, quote or paraphrase any part, or the content within this book, without the consent of the author or publisher.

Disclaimer Notice:

Please note the information contained within this document is for educational and entertainment purposes only. All effort has been executed to present accurate, up to date, and reliable, complete information. No warranties of any kind are declared or implied. Readers acknowledge that the author is not engaging in the rendering of legal, financial, medical or professional advice. The content within this book has been derived from various sources. Please consult a licensed professional before attempting any techniques outlined in this book.

By reading this document, the reader agrees that under no circumstances is the author responsible for any losses, direct or indirect, which are incurred as a result of the use of information contained within this document, including, but not limited to, — errors, omissions, or inaccuracies.

Table of contents

GREAT MEDITERRANEAN DIET RECIPES 6
   Italian Herb Bread 6
   Sumac Chickpea Bowl 8
   Smoked Salmon And Lemon-dill Ricotta Bento Box 11
   Mediterranean Baked Tilapia With Roasted Baby Red Potatoes 13
   Mediterranean Focaccia 15
   Cheesy Olive Bread 17
   Red Wine–marinated Flank Steak With Brussels Sprout Slaw 19
   One-pot Spanish Chicken Sausage And Shrimp With Rice 21
   Broccoli, Roasted Red Pepper, Cheddar, And Olive Frittata 23
   Chutney-dijon Pork Tenderloin With Mushroom And Kale Farro Pilaf 25
   Black Olive Bread 28
   Crispbread With Mascarpone And Berry-chia Jam 30
   Spiced Chicken-stuffed Zucchini With Brown Rice And Lentils 32
   Apple, Cinnamon, And Walnut Baked Oatmeal 35
   Chocolate–peanut Butter Yogurt With Berries 37
   Olive Fougasse 38
   Banana, Orange, And Pistachio Smoothie 40
   Breakfast Bento Box 41
   Maple-cardamom Chia Pudding With Blueberries 42
   Carrot-chickpea Fritters 43
   Whole-wheat Pasta With Lentil Bolognese 45
   Strawberries With Cottage Cheese And Pistachios 47
   Popcorn Trail Mix 48
   Creamy Shrimp-stuffed Portobello Mushrooms 49
   Rosemary Edamame, Zucchini, And Sun-dried Tomatoes With Garlic-chive Quinoa 51
   Baby Kale, Fennel, And Green Apple Salad 53
   Roasted Za'atar Salmon With Peppers And Sweet Potatoes 55
   Mediterranean mini frittatas 57
   Caprese avocado toast 59
   Mediterranean strata 60
   Slow cooker Mediterranean egg casserole 62
   Sheet pan eggs and veggies 64
   Hummus toast 66
   Breakfast egg muffins 67
   Foul mudammas 69
   Tahini banana shakes 71
   Shakshuka 72
   Simple green juice 74
   Greek chicken gyro salad 75

TUSCAN TUNA AND WHITE BEAN SALAD	77
AVOCADO CAPRESE SALAD	78
CITRUS SHRIMP AND AVOCADO SALAD	79
EASY COUSCOUS WITH SUNDRIED TOMATO AND FETA	81
GARLICKY SWISS CHARD AND CHICKPEAS	83
ARUGULA SALAD WITH PESTO SHRIMP, PARMESAN, AND WHITE BEANS	84
CANTALOUPE AND MOZZARELLA CAPRESE SALAD	86
ARUGULA SALAD	87
GREEK PASTA SALAD WITH CUCUMBER AND ARTICHOKE HEARTS	88
QUINOA AND KALE PROTEIN POWER SALAD	90
WHOLE WHEAT GREEK PASTA SALAD	92
TOMATO AND HEARTS OF PALM SALAD	94
QUINOA TABBOULEH WITH CHICKPEAS	95
AUTUMN COUSCOUS SALAD	97
SLOW COOKER CHICKEN CACCIATORE	99
GREEK BAKED COD WITH LEMON AND GARLIC	101
MOROCCAN FISH	103
LEMON GARLIC SALMON	105
SHEET PAN CHICKEN AND VEGETABLES	107

Great Mediterranean Diet Recipes

Italian Herb Bread

Servings: 25

Cooking Time: 40 Minutes

Ingredients:

1 2/3 teaspoons active dry yeast

3½ cups all-purpose flour

2 1/4 cup rye flour

1 tablespoon salt

2 tablespoons olive oil

1 tablespoon flat-leaf parsley, finely chopped

10 sprigs fresh thyme leaves, stems removed

1 garlic clove, peeled and finely chopped

¼ cup black olives, pitted and chopped

3 green chilies, deseeded and chopped

¾ cup sun-dried tomatoes, drained and chopped

Directions:

Take a bowl of lukewarm water (temperature of 0 degrees F) and dissolve 1 and 2/3 cups of yeast.

Add flour, yeast water, and salt to another bowl.

Mix well to prepare the dough using a mixer or your hands.

Put the dough in a large, clean bowl and allow it to rest covered for 2 hours.

Transfer dough to a lightly floured surface and knead, adding the parsley, garlic, olives, thyme, tomatoes, and chilies.

Place the kneaded dough in an 8½-inch bread-proofing basket.

Cover and allow to rest for about 60 minutes.

Preheat oven to 400 degrees F.

Line a baking sheet with parchment paper.

Bake for about 30-40 minutes.

Once done, enjoy it!

Nutrition Info: Calories: 338, Total Fat: 2.5 g, Saturated Fat: 0.4 g, Cholesterol: 0 mg, Sodium: 294 mg, Total Carbohydrate: 68.6 g, Dietary Fiber: 5.5 g, Total Sugars: 0.5 g, Protein: 10 g, Vitamin D: 0 mcg, Calcium: 53 mg, Iron: 7 mg, Potassium: 202 mg

Sumac Chickpea Bowl

Servings: 4
Cooking Time: 25 Minutes

Ingredients:
⅔ cup uncooked bulgur
1⅓ cups water
⅛ teaspoon kosher salt
1 teaspoon olive oil
2 tablespoons olive oil
2 (15.5-ounce) cans low-sodium chickpeas, drained and rinsed
3 tablespoons sumac
¼ teaspoon kosher salt
4 Persian cucumbers, quartered lengthwise and chopped (about 2 cups)
10 ounces cherry tomatoes, quartered (halved if you have small tomatoes)
¼ cup chopped fresh mint
1 cup chopped fresh parsley
4 teaspoons olive oil
2 tablespoons plus 2 teaspoons freshly squeezed lemon juice
¼ teaspoon kosher salt
2 tablespoons unsalted tahini
¼ teaspoon garlic powder
5 tablespoons water

Directions:

TO MAKE THE BULGUR

Place the bulgur, water, and salt in a saucepan, and bring to a boil. Once it boils, cover the pot with a lid and turn off the heat. Let the covered pot stand for minutes. Stir the oil into the cooked bulgur. Cool.

Place ½ cup of bulgur in each of 4 microwaveable containers.

TO MAKE THE CHICKPEAS

Heat the oil in a 12-inch skillet over medium-high heat. Once the oil is shimmering, add the chickpeas, sumac, and salt, and stir to coat. Cook for 2 minutes without stirring. Give the chickpeas a stir and cook for another 2 minutes without stirring. Stir and cook for 2 more minutes.

Place ¾ cup of cooled chickpeas in each of the 4 bulgur containers.

TO MAKE THE SALAD

Combine all the ingredients for the salad in a medium mixing bowl. Taste for salt and lemon, and add more if you need it.

Place 1¼ cup of salad in each of 4 containers. These containers will not be reheated.

TO MAKE THE TAHINI SAUCE

Combine the tahini and garlic powder in a small bowl. Whisk in 1 tablespoon of water at a time until all 5 tablespoons have been incorporated and a thin sauce has formed. It will thicken as it sits.

Place 1 tablespoon of tahini sauce in each of 4 small sauce containers.

STORAGE: Store covered containers in the refrigerator for up to 5 days. When serving, reheat the bulgur and chickpeas, add them to the salad, and drizzle the tahini sauce over the top.

Nutrition Info: Total calories: 485; Total fat: 19g; Saturated fat: 2g; Sodium: 361mg; Carbohydrates: 67g; Fiber: 19g; Protein: 16g

Smoked Salmon And Lemon-dill Ricotta Bento Box

Servings: 4

Cooking Time: 10 Minutes

Ingredients:

FOR THE LEMON-DILL RICOTTA

1 (16-ounce) container whole-milk ricotta cheese

1 teaspoon finely grated lemon zest

3 tablespoons chopped fresh dill

FOR THE BENTO BOX

8 ounces smoked salmon

4 (6-inch) Persian cucumbers or 2 small European cucumbers, sliced

2 cups sugar snap peas

4 whole-wheat pitas, each cut into 4 pieces

Directions:

Mix all the ingredients for the lemon-dill ricotta in a medium bowl.

Divide the salmon, cucumbers, and snap peas among 4 containers.

Place 1 pita in each of 4 resealable bags.

Place ½ cup of ricotta spread in each of separate small containers, since it may release some liquid after a couple of days.

STORAGE: Store covered containers in the refrigerator for up to 4 days. Store the pita at room temperature or in the refrigerator.

Nutrition Info: Total calories: 4; Total fat: 20g; Saturated fat: 11g; Sodium: 1,388mg; Carbohydrates: 40g; Fiber: 8g; Protein: 32g

Mediterranean Baked Tilapia With Roasted Baby Red Potatoes

Servings: 2

Cooking Time: 35 Minutes

Ingredients:

3 teaspoons olive oil, divided

1 small yellow onion, very thinly sliced (about 2½ cups)

1 large red bell pepper, thinly sliced (about 2 cups)

10 ounces baby red potatoes, quartered (about 1-inch pieces)

⅜ teaspoon kosher salt, divided

1 teaspoon chopped garlic

1 tablespoon capers, drained, rinsed, and roughly chopped

¼ cup golden raisins

1 (½-ounce) pack fresh basil, roughly chopped

2½ ounces baby spinach, large leaves torn in half (about 4 cups)

2 teaspoons freshly squeezed lemon juice

8 ounces tilapia or other thin white fish (see tip)

Directions:

Preheat the oven to 450°F. Line a sheet pan with a silicone baking mat or parchment paper.

Heat teaspoons of oil in a 12-inch skillet over medium heat. When the oil is shimmering, add the onions and peppers. Cook for 12 minutes, stirring occasionally. The onions should be very soft.

While the onions and peppers are cooking, place the potatoes on the sheet pan and toss with ⅛ teaspoon of salt and the remaining 1 teaspoon of oil. Spread the potatoes out evenly across half of the pan. Roast in the oven for 10 minutes.

Once the onions are soft, add the garlic, capers, raisins, basil, ⅛ teaspoon of salt, and the spinach. Stir to combine and cook for 3 more minutes to wilt the spinach.

Carefully remove the sheet pan from the oven after 10 minutes. Add half of the onion mixture to the empty side of the pan to form a nest for the fish. Place the fish on top and season with the remaining ⅛ teaspoon of salt and the lemon juice. Spread the rest of the onion mixture evenly across the top of the fish.

Place the pan back in the oven and cook for 10 minutes. The fish should be flaky.

When the fish and potatoes have cooled, place 1 piece of fish plus half of the potatoes and half of the onion mixture in each of 2 containers. Refrigerate.

STORAGE: Store covered containers in the refrigerator for up to 4 days.

Nutrition Info: Total calories: 427; Total fat: ; Saturated fat: 2g; Sodium: 952mg; Carbohydrates: 59g; Fiber: 10g; Protein: 31g

Mediterranean Focaccia

Servings: 4
Cooking Time: 30 Minutes

Ingredients:
3 3/5 cups flour
1 1/7 cups warm water
2 tablespoons olive oil
2 teaspoons dry yeast
1½ teaspoons salt
1 cup black olives, pitted and coarsely chopped
sea salt
olive oil

Directions:
Place flour and yeast in a large bowl.
Make a well and pour in water, salt, and oil.
Gradually keep mixing until everything is incorporated well.
Knead for about 20 minutes.
Add black olives and mix well.
Form a ball and allow it to rise for about 45 minutes (in a bowl covered with a towel).
Once the dough is ready, push air out of it by crushing it using your palm.
Roll out the dough onto a floured surface to a thickness of about ½ an inch.

Place it on a baking sheet covered with parchment paper, and allow the dough to rise for another 45 minutes.

Preheat oven to 425 degrees Fahrenheit.

Press fingers into the dough at regular intervals to pierce the dough.

When ready to bake, pour a bit of olive oil into the holes and sprinkle with salt.

Bake for 20-30 minutes.

Enjoy!

Nutrition Info: Calories: 523, Total Fat: 11.7 g, Saturated Fat: 1.7 g, Cholesterol: 0 mg, Sodium: 3495 mg, Total Carbohydrate: 89.4 g, Dietary Fiber: 4.6 g, Total Sugars: 0.3 g, Protein: 13.8 g, Vitamin D: 0 mcg, Calcium: 50 mg, Iron: 7 mg, Potassium: 124 mg

Cheesy Olive Bread

Servings: 8

Cooking Time: 15 Minutes

Ingredients:

½ cup softened butter

¼ cup mayo

1 teaspoon garlic powder

1 teaspoon onion powder

2 cups shredded mozzarella cheese

½ cup chopped black olives

1 loaf of French Bread, halved longways

Directions:

Preheat oven to a temperature of 350 degrees Fahrenheit.

Stir butter and mayo together in a bowl until it is smooth and creamy.

Add onion powder, garlic powder, olives, and cheese and stir.

Spread the mixture over French bread.

Place bread on a baking sheet and bake for 10-12 minutes.

Increase the heat to broil and cook until the cheese has melted and the bread is golden brown.

Cool and chill.

Pre-heat before eating.

Nutrition Info: Calories: 307, Total Fat: 17.7 g, Saturated Fat: 2 g, Cholesterol: 38 mg, Sodium: 482 mg, Total Carbohydrate: 30.1 g, Dietary Fiber: 1.5 g, Total Sugars: 1.9 g, Protein: 8 g, Vitamin D: 0 mcg, Calcium: 40 mg, Iron: 2 mg, Potassium: 73 mg

Red Wine–marinated Flank Steak With Brussels Sprout Slaw

Servings: 2

Cooking Time: 10 Minutes

Ingredients:

FOR THE STEAK

8 ounces flank steak, trimmed of visible fat

½ cup red wine

2 tablespoons low-sodium soy sauce

1 tablespoon olive oil

½ teaspoon garlic powder

FOR THE BRUSSELS SPROUT SLAW

8 ounces Brussels sprouts, stemmed, halved, and very thinly sliced

3 tablespoons unsalted sunflower seeds

3 tablespoons freshly squeezed lemon juice

1 tablespoon plus 1 teaspoon olive oil

2 tablespoons dried cranberries

⅛ teaspoon kosher salt

⅔ cup Artichoke-Olive Compote

Directions:

TO MAKE THE STEAK

Place all the ingredients for the steak in a gallon-size resealable bag. Allow the steak to marinate overnight or up to hours.

Place the oven rack about 6 inches from the heating element. Preheat the oven to the broil setting (use the high setting if you have multiple settings).

Cover a sheet pan with foil. Lift the steak out of the marinade and place on top of the foil-lined sheet pan. Place the pan in the oven and cook for to 6 minutes on one side. Flip the steak over to the other side and broil for 4 to 6 minutes more.

Remove from the oven and allow to rest for to 10 minutes. Medium-rare will be about 135°F when an instant-read meat thermometer is inserted.

On a cutting board, slice the steak thinly against the grain and divide the steak between 2 containers.

TO MAKE THE BRUSSELS SPROUT SLAW

Combine the Brussels sprouts, sunflower seeds, lemon juice, olive oil, cranberries, and salt in a medium bowl.

Place 1 cup of Brussels sprout slaw and ⅓ cup of artichoke-olive compote in each of 2 containers. The slaw and compote are meant to be eaten at room temperature, while the steak can be eaten warm. However, if you want to eat the steak at room temperature as well, all the items can be put in the same container.

STORAGE: Store covered containers in the refrigerator for up to 5 days.

Nutrition Info: Total calories: 601; Total fat: 31g; Saturated fat: 3g; Sodium: 1,098mg; Carbohydrates: 26g; Fiber: 5g; Protein: 29g

One-pot Spanish Chicken Sausage And Shrimp With Rice

Servings: 4

Cooking Time: 30 Minutes

Ingredients:

4 teaspoons olive oil, divided

1 (12-ounce) package cooked chicken sausage, sliced

6 ounces uncooked peeled, deveined medium shrimp

1 large green bell pepper, chopped (about 1½ cups)

1 small yellow onion, chopped (about 2 cups)

2 teaspoons chopped garlic

2 teaspoons smoked paprika

1 teaspoon dried thyme leaves

1 teaspoon dried oregano

½ teaspoon kosher salt

½ cup quick-cooking or instant brown rice

1 (14.5-ounce) can no-salt-added diced tomatoes in juice

1 cup low-sodium chicken broth

1 medium zucchini, halved vertically and sliced into half-moons

Directions:

Heat 2 teaspoons of oil in a soup pot over medium-high heat. When the oil is shimmering, add the sausage and brown for 5 minutes. Add the shrimp and cook for more minute. Remove the sausage and shrimp, and place them on a plate.

Add the remaining teaspoons of oil to the pot, and when the oil is shimmering, add the bell pepper, onion, and garlic. Sauté until soft, about 5 minutes.

Add the sausage, shrimp, paprika, thyme, oregano, salt, rice, tomatoes, and broth to the pot, and stir to combine. Bring to a boil, then cover the pot and turn the heat down to low. Simmer for 15 minutes.

After 15 minutes, add the zucchini, return the cover to the pot, and continue to simmer for 5 to 10 more minutes, until the zucchini is crisp-tender and the rice has absorbed most of the liquid.

Place about 2 cups of the rice mixture in each of 4 containers.

STORAGE: Store covered containers in the refrigerator for up to 5 days.

Nutrition Info: Total calories: 333; Total fat: 14g; Saturated fat: 3g; Sodium: 954mg; Carbohydrates: 29g; Fiber: 6g; Protein: 26g

Broccoli, Roasted Red Pepper, Cheddar, And Olive Frittata

Servings: 5

Cooking Time: 25 Minutes

Ingredients:

Oil or cooking spray for greasing the pan

8 large eggs

½ cup low-fat (2%) milk

1 teaspoon smoked paprika

6 ounces broccoli florets, finely chopped (about 2 cups)

½ cup chopped jarred roasted red peppers, drained of liquid

⅓ cup pitted black olives, chopped (or other olive of your choice)

¼ cup shredded sharp Cheddar cheese, plus 2 tablespoons

Directions:

Preheat the oven to 375°F and rub an 8-inch round cake or pie pan with oil, or spray with cooking spray.

Break the eggs into a large mixing bowl. Add the milk and smoked paprika, and whisk until well combined.

Add the chopped broccoli, red peppers, olives, and ¼ cup of cheese, and mix.

Pour the mixture into the oiled pan and top with the remaining 2 tablespoons of cheese. Bake for 20 to 25 minutes.

Once the frittata is cool, run a spatula around the sides and slice into pieces.

Place 1 slice in each of 5 containers and refrigerate.

STORAGE: Store covered containers in the refrigerator for up to 5 days.

Nutrition Info: Total calories: 193; Total fat: 12g; Saturated fat: 5g; Sodium: 295mg; Carbohydrates: 7g; Fiber: 1g; Protein: 13g

Chutney-dijon Pork Tenderloin With Mushroom And Kale Farro Pilaf

Servings: 2

Cooking Time: 40 Minutes

Ingredients:

8 ounces pork tenderloin (freeze half if you can only find a 1-pound package)

⅓ cup prepared mango or apricot chutney, plus 1 tablespoon

2 tablespoons Dijon mustard

1 teaspoon chopped garlic

2 teaspoons olive oil

2 teaspoons olive oil

4 ounces mushrooms, sliced

1 small bunch (about 7 ounces) lacinato or curly kale, ribs removed, leaves roughly chopped

½ teaspoon chopped garlic

⅔ cup farro

¼ cup dry red wine, such as red zinfandel, merlot, or cabernet

1¼ cups low-sodium vegetable broth (or chicken broth)

¼ teaspoon kosher salt

Directions:

TO MAKE THE PORK

Remove the tough silver skin from the tenderloin with a sharp knife.

In a small bowl, combine ⅓ cup of chutney and the mustard, garlic, and oil.

Place the pork in a gallon-size resealable bag or shallow dish and rub the chutney mixture over the pork. Marinate for at least 8 hours.

When you're ready to cook, preheat the oven to 0°F and line a sheet pan with a silicone baking mat or foil.

Remove the pork from the marinade and place it on the sheet pan. Discard the marinade. Place the pork in the oven for 10 minutes. Turn it over, rub the remaining 1 tablespoon of chutney over the top and sides, and roast for another 8 minutes. (Don't worry if extra marinade burns on the baking mat. The pork will be okay.)

Let the pork cool for at least 10 minutes and slice.

Divide the slices between 2 containers.

TO MAKE THE MUSHROOM AND KALE FARRO PILAF

Heat the oil in a soup pot or Dutch oven over medium-high heat. When the oil is shimmering, add the mushrooms and cook for 4 minutes.

Add the kale and garlic, stir, and cook for another 5 minutes.

Add the farro, stir, and cook for 1 minute. Add the red wine and allow to cook for 1 more minute.

Add the broth and salt, increase the heat to high, and bring to a boil. Once it is boiling, turn the heat down to low, cover, and simmer for 30 minutes, until the farro is tender but still has some bite to it.

After it has cooled, place 1 heaping cup of pilaf in each of the 2 pork containers. Refrigerate.

STORAGE: Store covered containers in the refrigerator for up to 5 days. Freeze farro pilaf for up to 6 months.

Nutrition Info: Total calories: 677; Total fat: 18g; Saturated fat: 3g; Sodium: 1,041mg; Carbohydrates: 76g; Fiber: 10g; Protein: 48g

Black Olive Bread

Servings: 6
Cooking Time: 45 Minutes

Ingredients:

3 cups bread flour
2 teaspoons active dry yeast
2 tablespoons white sugar
1 teaspoon salt
½ cup black olives, chopped
3 tablespoons olive oil
1¼ cups warm water (about 110 degrees Fahrenheit)
1 tablespoon cornmeal

Directions:

In a large bowl, combine flour, sugar, yeast, salt, black olives, water, and olive oil.
Mix well to prepare the dough.
Turn the dough onto a floured surface and knead well for 5-10 minutes until elastic.
Set dough aside and allow it to rise for about minutes until it has doubled in size.
Punch the dough down and knead again for 10 minutes.
Allow it to rise for 30 minutes more.
Round up the dough on a kneading board, place upside down in a bowl, and line it with a lint-free, well-floured towel.

Allow it to rise until it has doubled in size again.

While the bread is rising up for the third and final time, take a pan, fill it up with water, and place it at the bottom of your oven. Preheat oven to a temperature of 500 degrees Fahrenheit.

Turn the loaf out onto a sheet pan, lightly oil it, and dust with cornmeal.

Bake for about 15 minutes.

Reduce heat to 375 degrees Fahrenheit and bake for another 30 minutes.

Cool and chill.

Enjoy!

Nutrition Info: Calories: 324, Total Fat: 8.9 g, Saturated Fat: 1.3 g, Cholesterol: 0 mg, Sodium: 488 mg, Total Carbohydrate: 53.9 g, Dietary Fiber: 2.4 g, Total Sugars: 4.2 g, Protein: 7.2 g, Vitamin D: 0 mcg, Calcium: 20 mg, Iron: 4 mg, Potassium: 98 mg

Crispbread With Mascarpone And Berry-chia Jam

Servings: 3

Cooking Time: 5 Minutes

Ingredients:

- 1 (1-pound) bag frozen mixed berries
- 2 teaspoons freshly squeezed lemon juice
- 2 teaspoons pure maple syrup
- 2 tablespoons plus 2 teaspoons chia seeds
- 6 slices crispbread
- 3 tablespoons mascarpone cheese

Directions:

Place the frozen berries in a saucepan over medium heat. When the berries are defrosted, about 5 minutes, mash with a potato masher. You can leave them chunky.

Turn the heat off and add the lemon juice, maple syrup, and chia seeds.

Allow the jam to cool, then place in the refrigerator to thicken for about an hour.

Place 2 slices of crispbread in each of 3 resealable sandwich bags. Place 1 tablespoon of mascarpone and 2 tablespoons of jam in each of 3 containers with dividers. Alternatively, put the mascarpone and jam in separate small sauce containers.

STORAGE: Store crispbread at room temperature and jam and mascarpone in the refrigerator. Mascarpone will last for 7 days in the refrigerator, while jam will last for 2 weeks. Jam can be frozen for up to 3 months.

Nutrition Info: Total calories: 2; Total fat: 9g; Saturated fat: 3g; Sodium: 105mg; Carbohydrates: 40g; Fiber: 14g; Protein: 6g

Spiced Chicken-stuffed Zucchini With Brown Rice And Lentils

Servings: 3

Cooking Time: 35 Minutes

Ingredients:

⅓ cup long-grain brown rice

1⅔ cups water

⅛ teaspoon kosher salt

⅓ cup brown lentils

2 teaspoons olive oil

3 tablespoons chopped fresh dill

3 medium zucchini, halved lengthwise and flesh scooped out with a teaspoon (zucchini flesh reserved)

3 teaspoons olive oil, divided

1 small yellow onion, chopped

1 teaspoon chopped garlic

½ pound ground lean chicken

¾ teaspoon ground cumin

¾ teaspoon ground coriander

¾ teaspoon caraway seeds

⅛ teaspoon red chili flakes

3 tablespoons tomato paste

¼ teaspoon kosher salt

¼ cup feta cheese

Directions:

TO MAKE THE BROWN RICE AND LENTILS

Place the rice, water, and salt in a saucepan over high heat. Once the water is boiling, cover the pan and reduce the heat to low. Simmer for 15 minutes.

After 15 minutes, add the lentils and stir. Cover the pan and cook for another 15 minutes.

If there is a little bit of water still in the pan after the rice and lentils are tender, cook uncovered for a couple of minutes.

Stir in the oil and chopped dill.

Once the mixture has cooled, place ⅔ cup in each of 3 containers.

TO MAKE THE STUFFED ZUCCHINI

Preheat the oven to 400°F and line a sheet pan with a silicone baking mat or parchment paper. Place the zucchini boats on a lined sheet pan and coat with 1 teaspoon of oil.

In a 12-inch skillet, heat the remaining 2 teaspoons of oil over medium-high heat. When the oil is shimmering, add the onion and garlic and cook for 5 minutes. Add the zucchini flesh and cook for 2 more minutes.

Add the ground chicken, breaking it up with a spatula. Cook for 5 more minutes.

Add the cumin, coriander, caraway seeds, chili flakes, tomato paste, and salt, and cook for another 2 minutes.

Mound the chicken mixture into the zucchini boats. Top each zucchini boat with 2 teaspoons of feta cheese. Bake for 20 minutes.

Once cooled, place 2 zucchini halves in each of the 3 rice-and-lentil containers.

STORAGE: Store covered containers in the refrigerator for up to 5 days. Brown rice and lentils can be frozen for up to 3 months.

Nutrition Info: Total calories: 414; Total fat: 19g; Saturated fat: 5g; Sodium: 645mg; Carbohydrates: 39g; Fiber: 10g; Protein: 26g

Apple, Cinnamon, And Walnut Baked Oatmeal

Servings: 8

Cooking Time: 40 Minutes

Ingredients:

Cooking spray or oil for greasing the pan

3 small Granny Smith apples (about 1 pound), skin-on, chopped into ½-inch dice

3 cups rolled oats

1 teaspoon baking powder

3 tablespoons ground flaxseed

1 teaspoon ground cinnamon

2 eggs

¼ cup olive oil

1½ cups low-fat (2%) milk

⅓ cup pure maple syrup

½ cup walnut pieces (if you buy walnut halves, roughly chop the nuts)

Directions:

Preheat the oven to 350°F and spray an 8-by--inch baking dish with cooking spray or rub with oil.

Combine the apples, oats, baking powder, flaxseed, cinnamon, eggs, oil, milk, and maple syrup in a large mixing bowl and pour into the prepared baking dish.

Sprinkle the walnut pieces evenly across the oatmeal and bake for 40 minutes.

Allow the oatmeal to cool and cut it into 8 pieces. Place 1 piece in each of 5 containers. Take the other 3 pieces and either eat as a snack during the week or freeze for a later time.

STORAGE: Store covered containers in the refrigerator for up to 6 days. If frozen, oatmeal will last 6 months.

Nutrition Info: Total calories: 349; Total fat: 18g; Saturated fat: 3g; Sodium: 108mg; Carbohydrates: 43g; Fiber: ; Protein: 9g

Chocolate–peanut Butter Yogurt With Berries

Servings: 4

Cooking Time: 15 Minutes

Ingredients:

2 cups low-fat (2%) plain Greek yogurt

4 tablespoons unsweetened cocoa powder

4 tablespoons natural-style peanut butter

1 tablespoon pure maple syrup

1 cup fresh or frozen berries of your choice

Directions:

In a medium bowl, mix the yogurt, cocoa powder, peanut butter, and maple syrup until well combined.

Spoon ½ cup of the yogurt mixture and ¼ cup of berries into each of 4 containers.

STORAGE: Store covered containers in the refrigerator for up to 5 days.

Nutrition Info: Total calories: 225; Total fat: 12g; Saturated fat: ; Sodium: 130mg; Carbohydrates: 19g; Fiber: 4g; Protein: 16g

Olive Fougasse

Servings: 4
Cooking Time: 20 Minutes

Ingredients:

3 2/3 cups bread flour
3 1/2 tablespoons olive oil
1 2/3 tablespoons bread yeast
1 1/4 cups black olives, chopped
1 teaspoon oregano
1 teaspoon salt
1 cup water

Directions:
Add flour to a bowl.
Make a well in the center and add the water and remaining Ingredients:.
Knead the dough well until it becomes slightly elastic.
Mold it into a ball and let stand for about 1 hour.
Divide the pastry into four pieces of equal portions.
Flatten the balls using a rolling pin and place it on a floured baking tray.
Make incisions on the bread.
Allow them to rest for about 30 minutes
Preheat oven to 425 degrees Fahrenheit.

Brush the Fougasse with olive oil and allow it to bake for 20 minutes.

Turn the oven off and allow it to rest for 5 minutes.

Remove and allow it to cool.

Enjoy!

Nutrition Info: Calories: 586, Total Fat: 18.1 g, Saturated Fat: 2.6 g, Cholesterol: 0 mg, Sodium: 371 mg, Total Carbohydrate: 92.2 g, Dietary Fiber: 5.6 g, Total Sugars: 0.3 g, Protein: 2 g, Vitamin D: 0 mcg, Calcium: 63 mg, Iron: 8 mg, Potassium: 232 mg

Banana, Orange, And Pistachio Smoothie

Servings: 3

Cooking Time: 25 Minutes

Ingredients:

1 (17.6-ounce) container plain low-fat (2%) Greek yogurt

3 very ripe medium bananas

1½ cups orange juice

¾ cup unsalted shelled pistachios

Directions:

Place all the ingredients in a blender and blend until smooth.

Pour 1¾ cups of the smoothie into each of 3 smoothie containers.

STORAGE: Store covered containers in the refrigerator for up to 4 days.

Nutrition Info: calories: 9; Total fat: 19g; Saturated fat: 4g; Sodium: 71mg; Carbohydrates: 55g; Fiber: 3g; Protein: 26g

Breakfast Bento Box

Servings: 2
Cooking Time: 12 Minutes

Ingredients:

2 eggs
2 ounces sliced prosciutto
20 small whole-grain crackers
20 whole, unsalted almonds (about ¼ cup)
2 (6-inch) Persian cucumbers, sliced
1 large pear, sliced

Directions:

Place the eggs in a saucepan and cover with water. Bring the water to a boil. As soon as the water starts to boil, place a lid on the pan and turn the heat off. Set a timer for minutes.
When the timer goes off, drain the hot water and run cold water over the eggs to cool. Peel the eggs when cool and cut in half.
Place 2 egg halves and half of the prosciutto, crackers, almonds, cucumber slices, and pear slices in each of 2 containers.
STORAGE: Store covered containers in the refrigerator for up to 5 days.

Nutrition Info: Total calories: 370; Total fat: 20g; Saturated fat: ; Sodium: 941mg; Carbohydrates: 35g; Fiber: 7g; Protein: 16g

Maple-cardamom Chia Pudding With Blueberries

Servings: 5

Cooking Time: 5 Minutes

Ingredients:

2½ cups low-fat (2%) milk

½ cup chia seeds

1 tablespoon plus 1 teaspoon pure maple syrup

¼ teaspoon ground cardamom

2½ cups frozen blueberries

Directions:

Place the milk, chia seeds, maple syrup, and cardamom in a large bowl and stir to combine.

Spoon ½ cup of the mixture into each of 5 containers.

Place ½ cup of frozen blueberries in each container and stir to combine. Let the pudding sit for at least an hour in the refrigerator before eating.

STORAGE: Store covered containers in the refrigerator for up to 5 days.

Nutrition Info: Total calories: 218; Total fat: 8g; Saturated fat: 2g; Sodium: 74mg; Carbohydrates: 28g; Fiber: 10g; Protein: 10g

Carrot-chickpea Fritters

Servings: 3

Cooking Time: 10 Minutes

Ingredients:

2 teaspoons olive oil, plus 1 tablespoon

3 cups shredded carrots

1 (4-ounce) bunch scallions, white and green parts chopped

1 (15-ounce) can low-sodium chickpeas, drained and rinsed

⅓ cup dried apricots (about 10 small apricot halves), chopped

1 teaspoon garlic powder

1½ teaspoons dried mint

⅓ cup chickpea flour

1 egg

¼ teaspoon kosher salt

1 tablespoon freshly squeezed lemon juice

1 (5-ounce) package arugula

¾ cup Garlic Yogurt Sauce

Directions:

Heat 2 teaspoons of oil in a -inch skillet over medium-high heat. Once the oil is hot, add the carrots and scallions, and cook for 5 minutes. Allow to cool.

While the carrots are cooking, mash the chickpeas in a large mixing bowl with the bottom of a coffee mug. (I find a coffee mug works better than a potato masher.)

Add the apricots, garlic powder, mint, chickpea flour, egg, salt, lemon juice, and cooked carrot mixture to the bowl, and stir until well combined.

Form 6 patties and place them on a plate.

Heat the remaining 1 tablespoon of oil in the same skillet over medium-high heat. Once the oil is hot, add the patties. Cook for 3 minutes on each side, or until each side is browned.

Place 2 cooled fritters in each of 3 containers. Place about 2 cups of arugula in each of 3 other containers, and spoon ¼ cup Garlic Yogurt Sauce into each of 3 separate containers, or next to the arugula. The arugula and sauce are served at room temperature, while the fritters will be reheated.

STORAGE: Store covered containers in the refrigerator for up to 5 days. Uncooked patties can be frozen for 3 to 4 months.

Nutrition Info: Total calories: 461; Total fat: 17g; Saturated fat: 3g; Sodium: 393mg; Carbohydrates: 61g; Fiber: 15g; Protein: 21g

Whole-wheat Pasta With Lentil Bolognese

Servings: 4

Cooking Time: 55 Minutes

Ingredients:

2 tablespoons olive oil, divided

1 small yellow onion, chopped (about 2 cups)

1 tablespoon chopped garlic

2 medium carrots, peeled, halved vertically, and sliced (about 1¼ cup)

8 ounces button or cremini mushrooms, roughly chopped (about 4 cups)

1 teaspoon dried Italian herbs

2 tablespoons tomato paste

½ cup dry red wine

1 (28-ounce) can no-salt-added crushed tomatoes

2 cups water

1 cup uncooked brown lentils

½ teaspoon kosher salt

8 ounces dry whole-wheat penne pasta

¼ cup nutritional yeast

Directions:

Heat a soup pot on medium-high heat with tablespoon of oil. Once the oil is shimmering, add the onion and garlic, and cook for 2 minutes.

Add the carrots and mushrooms, then stir and cook for another 5 minutes.

Add the Italian herbs and tomato paste, stir to evenly incorporate, and cook for 5 more minutes, without stirring.

Add the wine and scrape up any bits from the bottom of the pan. Cook for 2 more minutes.

Add the tomatoes, water, lentils, and salt. Bring to a boil, then turn the heat down to low and simmer for 40 minutes.

While the sauce is cooking, cook the pasta according to the package directions, drain, and cool.

When the sauce is done simmering, stir in the remaining 1 tablespoon of oil and the nutritional yeast. Cool the sauce.

Combine 1 cup of cooked pasta and 1⅓ cups of sauce in each of 4 containers. Freeze the remaining sauce for a later meal.

STORAGE: Store covered containers in the refrigerator for up to 5 days.

Nutrition Info: Total calories: 570; Total fat: 9g; Saturated fat: 1g; Sodium: 435mg; Carbohydrates: 96g; Fiber: 17g; Protein: 27g

Strawberries With Cottage Cheese And Pistachios

Servings: 5

Cooking Time: 35 Minutes

Ingredients:

16 ounces low-fat cottage cheese

16 ounces strawberries, hulled and sliced

½ cup plus 2 tablespoons unsalted shelled pistachios

Directions:

Spoon ⅓ cup of cottage cheese into each of 5 containers.

Top each scoop of cottage cheese with ⅔ cup of strawberries and tablespoons of pistachios.

Refrigerate.

STORAGE: Store covered containers in the refrigerator for up to 5 days.

Nutrition Info: Total calories: 184; Total fat: 9g; Saturated fat: 2g; Sodium: 26g; Carbohydrates: 14g; Fiber: 4g; Protein: 15g

Popcorn Trail Mix

Servings: 5
Cooking Time: 35 Minutes

Ingredients:
12 dried apricot halves, quartered
⅔ cup whole, unsalted almonds
½ cup green pumpkin seeds (pepitas)
4 cups air-popped lightly salted popcorn

Directions:
Place the apricots, almonds, and pumpkin seeds in a medium bowl and toss with clean hands to evenly mix.

Scoop about ⅓ cup of the mixture into each of 5 containers or resealable sandwich bags. Place ¾ cup of popcorn in each of 5 separate containers or resealable bags. You will have one extra serving.

Mix the popcorn and the almond mixture together when it's time to eat. (The apricots make the popcorn stale quickly, which is why they're stored separately.)

STORAGE: Store covered containers or resealable bags at room temperature for up to 5 days.

Nutrition Info: Total calories: 244; Total fat: 16g; Saturated fat: 2g; Sodium: 48mg; Carbohydrates: 19g; Fiber: ; Protein: 10g

Creamy Shrimp-stuffed Portobello Mushrooms

Servings: 3
Cooking Time: 40 Minutes

Ingredients:

1 teaspoon olive oil, plus 2 tablespoons
6 portobello mushrooms, caps and stems separated and stems chopped
6 ounces broccoli florets, finely chopped (about 2 cups)
2 teaspoons chopped garlic
10 ounces uncooked peeled, deveined shrimp, thawed if frozen, roughly chopped
1 (14.5-ounce) can no-salt-added diced tomatoes
4 tablespoons roughly chopped fresh basil
½ cup mascarpone cheese
¼ cup panko bread crumbs
4 tablespoons grated Parmesan, divided
¼ teaspoon kosher salt

Directions:

Preheat the oven to 350°F. Line a sheet pan with a silicone baking mat or parchment paper.
Rub 1 teaspoon of oil over the bottom (stem side) of the mushroom caps and place on the lined sheet pan, stem-side up.

Heat the remaining 2 tablespoons of oil in a 12-inch skillet on medium-high heat. Once the oil is shimmering, add the chopped mushroom stems and broccoli, and sauté for 2 to minutes. Add the garlic and shrimp, and continue cooking for 2 more minutes. Add the tomatoes, basil, mascarpone, bread crumbs, 3 tablespoons of Parmesan, and the salt. Stir to combine and turn the heat off.

With the mushroom cap openings facing up, mound slightly less than 1 cup of filling into each mushroom. Top each with ½ teaspoon of the remaining Parmesan cheese.

Bake the mushrooms for 35 minutes.

Place 2 mushroom caps in each of 3 containers.

STORAGE: Store covered containers in the refrigerator for up to 4 days.

Nutrition Info: Total calories: 47 Total fat: 31g; Saturated fat: 10g; Sodium: 526mg; Carbohydrates: 26g; Fiber: 7g; Protein: 26g

Rosemary Edamame, Zucchini, And Sun-dried Tomatoes With Garlic-chive Quinoa

Servings: 4

Cooking Time: 15 Minutes

Ingredients:

FOR THE GARLIC-CHIVE QUINOA

1 teaspoon olive oil

1 teaspoon chopped garlic

⅔ cup quinoa

1⅓ cups water

¼ teaspoon kosher salt

1 (¾-ounce) package fresh chives, chopped

FOR THE ROSEMARY EDAMAME, ZUCCHINI, AND SUN-DRIED TOMATOES

1 teaspoon oil from sun-dried tomato jar

2 medium zucchini, cut in half lengthwise and sliced into half-moons (about 3 cups)

1 (12-ounce) package frozen shelled edamame, thawed (2 cups)

½ cup julienne-sliced sun-dried tomatoes in olive oil, drained

¼ teaspoon dried rosemary

⅛ teaspoon kosher salt

Directions:

TO MAKE THE GARLIC-CHIVE QUINOA

Heat the oil over medium heat in a saucepan. Once the oil is shimmering, add the garlic and cook for 1 minute, stirring often so it doesn't burn.

Add the quinoa and stir a few times. Add the water and salt and turn the heat up to high. Once the water is boiling, cover the pan and turn the heat down to low. Simmer the quinoa for 15 minutes, or until the water is absorbed.

Stir in the chives and fluff the quinoa with a fork.

Place ½ cup quinoa in each of 4 containers.

TO MAKE THE ROSEMARY EDAMAME, ZUCCHINI, AND SUN-DRIED TOMATOES

Heat the oil in a 12-inch skillet over medium-high heat. Once the oil is shimmering, add the zucchini and cook for 2 minutes.

Add the edamame, sun-dried tomatoes, rosemary, and salt, and cook for another 6 minutes, or until the zucchini is crisp-tender.

Spoon 1 cup of the edamame mixture into each of the 4 quinoa containers.

STORAGE: Store covered containers in the refrigerator for up to 5 days.

Nutrition Info: Total calories: 312; Total fat: ; Saturated fat: 1g; Sodium: 389mg; Carbohydrates: 39g; Fiber: 9g; Protein: 15g

Baby Kale, Fennel, And Green Apple Salad

Servings: 3

Cooking Time: 15 Minutes

Ingredients:

1 teaspoon olive oil

1 teaspoon chopped garlic

⅔ cup quinoa

1⅓ cups water

1 cooked rotisserie chicken, meat removed and shredded (about 9 ounces)

1 fennel bulb, core and fronds removed, thinly sliced (about 2 cups)

1 small green apple, julienned (about 1½ cups)

8 tablespoons Honey-Lemon Vinaigrette, divided

1 (5-ounce) package baby kale

6 tablespoons walnut pieces

Directions:

Heat the oil over medium heat in a saucepan. Once the oil is shimmering, add the garlic and cook for minute, stirring often so that it doesn't burn.

Add the quinoa and stir a few times. Add the water and turn the heat up to high. Once the water is boiling, cover the pan and turn the heat down to low. Simmer the quinoa for 15 minutes, or until the water is absorbed. Cool.

Place the chicken, fennel, apple, and cooled quinoa in a large bowl. Add 2 tablespoons of the vinaigrette to the bowl and mix to combine.

Divide the baby kale, chicken mixture, and walnuts among 3 containers. Pour 2 tablespoons of the remaining vinaigrette into each of 3 sauce containers.

STORAGE: Store covered containers in the refrigerator for up to days.

Nutrition Info: Total calories: 9; Total fat: 39g; Saturated fat: 6g; Sodium: 727mg; Carbohydrates: 49g; Fiber: 8g; Protein: 29g

Roasted Za'atar Salmon With Peppers And Sweet Potatoes

Servings: 4

Cooking Time: 25 Minutes

Ingredients:

FOR THE VEGGIES

2 large red bell peppers, cut into ½-inch strips

1 pound sweet potatoes, peeled and cut into 1-inch chunks

1 tablespoon olive oil

¼ teaspoon kosher salt

FOR THE SALMON

2¾ teaspoons sesame seeds

2¾ teaspoons dried thyme leaves

2¾ teaspoons sumac

1 pound skinless, boneless salmon fillet, divided into 4 pieces

⅛ teaspoon kosher salt

1 teaspoon olive oil

2 teaspoons freshly squeezed lemon juice

Directions:

TO MAKE THE VEGGIES

Preheat the oven to 4°F.

Place silicone baking mats or parchment paper on two sheet pans.

On the first pan, place the peppers and sweet potatoes. Pour the oil and sprinkle the salt over both and toss to coat. Spread everything out in an even layer. Place the sheet pan in the oven and set a timer for 10 minutes.

TO MAKE THE SALMON

Mix the sesame seeds, thyme, and sumac together in a small bowl to make the za'atar spice mix.

Place the salmon fillets on the second sheet pan. Sprinkle the salt evenly across the fillets. Spread ¼ teaspoon of oil and ½ teaspoon of lemon juice over each piece of salmon.

Pat 2 teaspoons of the za'atar spice mix over each piece of salmon.

When the veggie timer goes off, place the salmon in the oven with the veggies and bake for 10 minutes for salmon that is ½ inch thick and for 15 minutes for salmon that is 1 inch thick. The veggies should be done when the salmon is done cooking.

Place one quarter of the veggies and 1 piece of salmon in each of 4 separate containers.

STORAGE: Store covered containers in the refrigerator for up to 4 days.

Nutrition Info: Total calories: 295; Total fat: 10g; Saturated fat: 2g; Sodium: 249mg; Carbohydrates: 29g; Fiber: 6g; Protein: 25g

Mediterranean mini frittatas

Preparation time: 20 minutes
Cooking time: 25 minutes
Servings: 12

Ingredients:
¼ cup crumbled feta cheese
1 tsp olive oil
1 cup chopped mushrooms
1 cup sliced zucchini
1/3 cup diced red onion
¼ cup chopped Kalamata olives
2 cups spinach
½ tsp dried oregano
½ cup fat-free milk
Six eggs
Black pepper to taste

Directions:
Sauté mushrooms, zucchini, and onions for about two minutes in heated oil in a skillet over medium flame.
Mix spinach in the mushroom mixture after lowering the flame. Add oregano and olives.
Cook for two more minutes with occasional stirring. When spinach is done, remove the cooking skillet and set aside.
Mix pepper, eggs, cheese, milk, and sautéed veggies in a bowl.

In an oil muffin pan, pour egg/veggies mixture.

Bake in a preheated oven at 350 degrees for 20 minutes and serve.

Nutrition Info: Calories: 128 kcal Fat: 8 g Protein: 9 g Carbs: 4 g Fiber: 1 g

Caprese avocado toast

Preparation time: 10 minutes
Cooking time: 0 minute
Servings: 1

Ingredients:
Two avocados
¼ cup chopped basil leaves
2 tsp lemon juice
4 oz sliced mozzarella
Sea salt to taste
Four toasted slices of bread
Black pepper to taste
1 cup halved grape tomatoes
Balsamic glaze for drizzling

Directions: In a bowl, add sliced avocados, salt, lemon juice, and pepper and mix well.
Over medium flame, lightly toast the bread.
Using a knife, spread avocados mixture over bread slices.
Sprinkle salt, basil, cheese, pepper, balsamic glaze, and tomatoes.
Serve and enjoy it.

Nutrition Info: Calories: 338 kcal Fat: 20.4 g Protein: 12.8 g Carbs: 25.8 g Fiber: 9.2 g

Mediterranean strata

Preparation time: 20 minutes
Cooking time: 55 minutes
Servings: 7

Ingredients:
2 tbsp olive oil
One minced clove garlic
1/2 diced yellow onion
1 lb chicken sausage
1/2 cup halved Kalamata olives
6 cups white bread
1/2 cup chopped sun-dried tomatoes
1/4 cup chopped fresh basil
1/2 cup crumbled feta cheese
Eight eggs
Salt and pepper to taste
2 cups of milk
Red pepper flakes

Directions:
Heat butter and oil over medium flame in skillet. Sauté onions for two minutes. Stir in garlic and chicken sausage.
Cook until sausages are done.
Mix olives, cook sausages, onions, sun-dried tomatoes, pepper, bread, garlic, feta cheese, basil, red chili flakes, and salt.

Mix milk and egg in a small bowl and add in sausage mixture.

Pour the sausage mixture into the baking tray.

Bake in preheated oven for 50 minutes and serve after garnishing with basil.

Nutrition Info: Calories: 297 kcal Fat: 9.5 g Protein: 17.9 g Carbs: 36 g Fiber: 3.1 g

Slow cooker Mediterranean egg casserole

Preparation time: 25 minutes
Cooking time: 480 minutes
Servings: 10

Ingredients:

2 oz cut prosciutto
3 cups sliced cremini mushrooms
1 tbsp butter
1/2 chopped red pepper
10 oz chopped spinach
16 oz ORE-IDA Diced Hash Brown Potatoes
1 cup sliced artichoke hearts
8 oz cheddar & Swiss Cheese
1/4 cup chopped sun-dried tomato
4 oz goat cheese
1 tbsp Dijon Mustard
Eight eggs
fresh basil leaves for garnish
2 cups whole milk

Directions:

Sauté prosciutto for four minutes in a pan over medium flame. Set aside.
In the same pan, cook bell pepper and mushrooms in the melted butter.

Make layers of potatoes, bell pepper and mushroom mixture, spinach, sundried tomatoes, artichoke hearts, Swiss and cheddar cheese, and goat cheese in the slow cooker.

Mix mustard, milk, salt, eggs, and pepper spread over the veggie's layers in a slow cooker.

Spread prosciutto over the top and cook for about ten minutes on low flame.

Sprinkle basil and serve.

Nutrition Info: Calories: 310 kcal Fat: 19 g Protein: 18 g Carbs: 14 g Fiber: 3 g

Sheet pan eggs and veggies

Preparation time: 10 minutes
Cooking time: 15 minutes
Servings: 6

Ingredients:
One sliced bell pepper (green, red, and orange)
One sliced red onion
Salt to taste
Black pepper to taste
2 tsp za'atar blend,
1 tsp ground cumin and
1 tsp Aleppo chili pepper
Extra virgin olive oil as required
Six eggs
A handful of Chopped fresh parsley
One diced Roma tomato
Crumbled feta cheese

Directions:
In a bowl, whisk bell peppers, onions, salt, zaatar, Aleppo chili, cumin, olive oil, and black pepper. Mix well.
Shift the bell pepper mixture over the baking pan.
Bake in a preheated oven at 400 degrees for 15 minutes.
Make holes in baked vegetable mixture and crack one egg in each hole.

Again, bake for eight minutes.

Sprinkle cheese, parsley, and tomatoes and serve.

Nutrition Info: Calories: 111 kcal Fat: 7.3 g Protein: 6.9 g Carbs: 4.5 g Fiber: 1.1 g

Hummus toast

Preparation time: 10 minutes
Cooking time: 0 minute
Servings: 4

Ingredients:
Hummus
Whole-grain bread seeded
Topping option 1
Sprouts
Sliced avocado
Black sesame seeds
Topping option 2
Za'atar spice
Roasted chickpeas
Topping option 3
Sunflower seeds
Pumpkin seeds
Hemp seeds
Sesame seeds

Directions: Spread hummus using a knife over toast and top with any of the topping options given in ingredients and serve.

Nutrition Info: Calories: 300 kcal Fat: 8 g Protein: 10 g Carbs: 24 g Fiber: 7 g

Breakfast egg muffins

Preparation time: 15 minutes
Cooking time: 20 minutes
Servings: 6

Ingredients:
Base
Salt to taste
12 eggs
2 tbsp chopped onion
Black pepper to taste
Tomato spinach mozzarella
Eight sliced cherry tomatoes
1/4 cup chopped spinach
1/4 cup grated mozzarella cheese
Bacon cheddar
1/4 cup grated cheddar cheese
1/4 cup chopped bacon
Garlic mushroom pepper
1/4 cup diced red capsicum
1/4 cup sliced brown mushrooms
1/4 tsp minced garlic powder
1 tbsp chopped parsley

Directions:
Mix onions, salt, eggs, and black pepper in a bowl.

Pour egg mixture in muffin cups greased with oil.

Use all three toppings to top each of the muffin cups.

Bake in a preheated oven at 350 degrees for twenty minutes.

Serve and enjoy it.

Nutrition Info: Calories: 82 kcal Fat: 5 g Protein: 6 g Carbs: 1 g Fiber: 1 g

Foul mudammas

Preparation time: 15 minutes

Cooking time: 10 minutes

Servings: 5

Ingredients:

Extra virgin olive oil

Kosher salt to taste

30 oz plain fava beans

1 tsp ground cumin

One lemon juice

1 cup chopped parsley

Two chopped hot peppers

One diced tomato

Two chopped garlic cloves

To serve

Warm pit bread

Green onions

Sliced cucumbers

Sliced tomatoes

Olives

Directions:

Pour half cup of water, salt, beans, and cumin in a pan over medium flame and cook.

When beans are done, mash them using a masher.

Lightly blend garlic, lemon juice, and hot peppers.

Transfer roughly blended hot pepper mixture over mashed beans.

Ass olive oil, parsley, hot pepper slices, and chopped tomatoes and serve with veggies or bread.

Nutrition Info: Calories: 142 kcal Fat: 1 g Protein: 10 g Carbs: 25 g Fiber: 10 g

Tahini banana shakes

Preparation time: 5 minutes
Cooking time: 0 minute
Servings: 3

Ingredients:
¼ cup ice, crushed
1 ½ cups almond milk
¼ cup tahini
4 Medjool dates
Two sliced bananas
One pinch of ground cinnamon

Directions:
Blend all the ingredients in the blender to obtain a creamy and smooth mixture.
Pour mixture in cups and serve after sprinkling cinnamon over the top.

Nutrition Info: Calories: 299 kcal Fat: 12.4 g Protein: 5.7 g Carbs: 47.7 g Fiber: 5.6 g

Shakshuka

Preparation time: 15 minutes
Cooking time: 20 minutes
Servings: 6

Ingredients:
1 tsp ground cumin
2 tbsp olive oil
One chopped red bell pepper
Six eggs
¼ tsp salt
Three minced cloves garlic
Ground black pepper to taste
2 tbsp tomato paste
½ tsp smoked paprika
¼ tsp red pepper flakes
2 tbsp chopped cilantro for garnish
½ cup feta cheese
One chopped yellow onion
28 oz fire-roasted tomatoes, crushed
Crusty bread for serving

Directions:
Heat oil in a skillet over medium flame and cook bell pepper, onions, and salt in it for six minutes with constant stirring.

After six minutes, stir in tomato paste, red pepper flakes, cumin, garlic, and paprika. Cook for another two minutes.

Add crushed tomatoes and cilantro to the onion mixture. Let it simmer.

Reduce the flame and simmer for five minutes.

Use salt and pepper to adjust the flavor.

Crack eggs in small well made at different areas using a spoon.

Pour tomato mixture over eggs to help them cook while staying intact.

Bake the skillet in a preheated oven at 375 degrees for 12 minutes.

Garnish with cilantro, flakes, and cheese and serve.

Nutrition Info: Calories: 216 kcal Fat: 12.8 g Protein: 11.2 g Carbs: 16.6 g Fiber: 4.4 g

Simple green juice

Preparation time: 15 minutes
Cooking time: 0 minute
Servings: 2

Ingredients:
5 oz kale
1 tsp crushed ginger
One apple
Five trimmed celery stalks
½ English cucumber
1 oz parsley

Directions:
Blend all the ingredients in the blender and pour into serving cups.

Nutrition Info: Calories: 92 kcal Fat: 0.8 g Protein: 2.8 g Carbs: 21 g Fiber: 6.2 g

Greek chicken gyro salad

Preparation time: 15 minutes
Cooking time: 7 minutes
Servings: 4

Ingredients:
Chicken
3 tsp dried oregano
2 tbsp olive oil
1 tbsp red wine vinegar
1.25 lb boneless chicken breasts
1 tsp ground black pepper
1 tbsp lemon juice
1 tsp Kosher salt
Salad
1 cup diced English cucumber
6 cups lettuce
1 cup feta cheese diced
1 cup diced tomatoes
1/2 cup diced red onions
1 cup crushed pita chips
Tzatziki Sauce
1 tbsp white wine vinegar
3/4 tsp Kosher salt
8 oz Greek yogurt
One minced clove garlic

2/3 cup grated English cucumber

1 tbsp lemon juice

3/4 tsp ground black pepper

2 tsp dried dill weed

One pinch of sugar

Directions:

Heat oil in a skillet and add chicken, salt, oregano, and black pepper. Cook for five minutes over medium flame.

Reduce the flame to low and add lemon juice and vinegar and simmer for five minutes.

Continue cooking until the chicken is done. Now, the chicken is ready and set aside.

Combine tomatoes, pita chips, chicken, lettuce, cucumber, and onions. Mix and set aside. The salad is ready.

In another bowl, whisk yogurt, cucumber, garlic, lemon juice, vinegar, dill, salt, pepper, and sugar. Mix well. The sauce is ready.

Now, pour the sauce over the salad and serve with cooked chicken.

Nutrition Info: Calories: 737 kcal Fat: 29 g Protein: 64 g Carbs: 54 g Fiber: 6 g

Tuscan tuna and white bean salad

Preparation time: 5 minutes
Cooking time: 0 minute
Servings: 2

Ingredients:
2 tbsp extra virgin olive oil
15 oz cannellini beans
4 cups spinach
5 oz white albacore
1/4 cup sliced olives
1/2 cup diced cherry tomatoes
One sliced red onion
1/2 lemon
Kosher salt to taste
1/4 cup feta cheese
Black pepper to taste

Directions: Combine white beans, olives, lemon juice, arugula, onions, tuna, olive oil, and tomatoes in a mixing bowl. Sprinkle pepper and salt and feta cheese and serve.

Nutrition Info: Calories: 436 kcal Fat: 22 g Protein: 30 g Carbs: 39 g Fiber: 12 g

Avocado Caprese salad

Preparation time: 5 minutes
Cooking time: 0 minute
Servings: 1

Ingredients:
1 cup sliced cherry tomatoes
1/4 cup basil leaves
1/2 cup mozzarella cheese balls
½ avocado
2 tsp extra virgin olive oil
Salt to taste
2 tsp balsamic vinegar
Black pepper to taste

Directions:
In a bowl, combine cheese, tomatoes, avocado, olive oil, salt, basil, vinegar, and black pepper.
Mix well and serve.

Nutrition Info: Calories: 456 kcal Fat: 37 g Protein: 17 g Carbs: 20 g Fiber: 9 g

Citrus shrimp and avocado salad

Preparation time: 5 minutes
Cooking time: 10 minutes
Servings: 3

Ingredients:
1 tbsp olive oil
1/2 cup lemon juice
1 cup of orange juice
1/2 tsp stone house seasoning
3 lb shrimp
2 tbsp chopped parsley
8 cups salad greens
1/2 cup citrus vinaigrette
1/2 sliced red onion
One sliced avocado

Directions:
In a bowl, mix orange juice, stone house seasoning, oil, and lemon juice.
Transfer the bowl mixture to the heated skillet. Cook for five minutes over medium flame.
Stir in shrimps and cook for five more minutes.
Sprinkle parsley and set aside. Citrus shrimps are ready.
Prepare the Citrus Vinaigrette Dressing as per the instruction given on the package.

In a bowl, whisk citrus vinaigrette until it emulsified. Mix salad greens, avocado, shrimps, and onion in a citrus vinaigrette. Serve and enjoy it.

Nutrition Info: Calories: 430 kcal Fat: 21 g Protein: 48 g Carbs: 12 g Fiber: 3 g

Easy couscous with sundried tomato and feta

Preparation time: 12 minutes

Cooking time: minutes

Servings: 6

Ingredients:

1.25 cups dried couscous

1 tsp powdered vegetable stock

1.25 cups boiled water

One chopped garlic clove

14 oz chickpeas

1 tsp coriander powder

½ cup chopped coriander

One chopped onion

½ cup chopped parsley

7 oz sun-dried tomato

One lemon zest

4 oz arugula lettuce

Black pepper

5 tbsp lemon juice

2 oz feta cheese

½ tsp black pepper

Salt to taste

Directions:

In a bowl, combine garlic, chickpeas, stock powder, couscous, and coriander.

Add hot water to the bowl and mix well. Cover the bowl and keep it aside for about five minutes.

Add sun-dried tomatoes, lemon juice, coriander, rocket, pepper, parsley, salt, onions, and lemon zest and toss well.

Sprinkle feta cheese and serve.

Nutrition Info: Calories: 260 kcal Fat: 9.2 g Protein: 10 g Carbs: 39 g Fiber: 5.8 g

Garlicky Swiss chard and chickpeas

Preparation time: 10 minutes
Cooking time: 10 minutes
Servings: 4

Ingredients:
1 cup chopped sundried tomatoes
1 tbsp olive oil Two minced garlic cloves One sliced shallot Two bunches of chopped Swiss chard
15 oz chickpeas One lemon
1/4 cup vegetable broth

Directions:
Cook shallot in heated oil over medium flame until they turned translucent.
After shallots are translucent, stir in garlic and cook for three minutes.
Mix chard and broth and cover, and let it simmer for a few minutes.
Add lemon juice, sundried tomatoes, lemon zest, and chickpeas and mix to combine. Cook for three minutes.
Serve and enjoy.

Nutrition Info: Calories: 519 kcal Fat: 9 g Protein: 14 g Carbs: 87 g Fiber: 10 g

Arugula salad with pesto shrimp, parmesan, and white beans

Preparation time: 35 minutes

Cooking time: 15 minutes

Servings: 3

Ingredients:

4 tbsp olive oil

1/2 lb raw shrimp Two minced cloves garlic

1/4 tsp ground black pepper

1/4 tsp salt

One pinch of red pepper flakes

1/4 cup pesto Genovese 2 cups cherry tomatoes

8 cups Arugula

1/8 cup grated parmesan cheese

1/2 lemon

1/2 cup white beans

Directions:

In a mixing bowl, add salt, chili flakes, olive oil, shrimp, and black pepper. Mix well and keep it aside for 30 minutes for enhanced flavor.

Heat olive oil in a skillet over a high flame. Cook shrimps in oil, two minutes from each side.

Lower the flame and stir in tomatoes and garlic. Cook for five more minutes with occasional stirring.

Shift cooked shrimps' mixture in a bowl and mix with pesto.

In a bowl, mix olive oil, arugula, and lemon juice. Add cheese, tomatoes, salt, beans, and black pepper. Mix well.

Serve arugula mixture with cooked shrimps.

Nutrition Info: Calories: 276 kcal Fat: 6.7 g Protein: 30 g Carbs: 23.3 g Fiber: 5.5 g

Cantaloupe and Mozzarella Caprese salad

Preparation time: 10 minutes
Cooking time: 0 minute
Servings: 8

Ingredients:
1 tbsp white wine vinegar sliced cantaloupes
Eight shredded prosciutto
8 oz mozzarella balls
¼ cup chopped basil leaves tbsp extra-virgin olive oil
¼ cup chopped mint leaves
Salt to taste
1.5 tbsp honey
Black pepper to taste

Directions: Take cantaloupe balls out of cantaloupe using melon baller and place in a bowl.
Add mozzarella cheese ball, prosciutto, basil, and mint leaves. Mix well.
In another bowl, mix honey, vinegar, and olive oil. Pour the dressing over a cantaloupe mixture and mix well.
Serve and enjoy it.

Nutrition Info: Calories: 232 kcal Fat: 15 g Protein: 10 g Carbs: 17 g Fiber: 2 g

Arugula salad

Preparation time: 5 minutes
Cooking time: 0 minute
Servings: 2

Ingredients:
4 cups arugula tbsp olive oil
1/2 tsp kosher salt tbsp lemon juice
1/2 tsp black pepper
1/4 cup grated parmesan cheese
1 tsp honey

Directions:
Combine honey, black pepper, parmesan cheese, olive oil, salt, arugula, and lemon juice. Toss to coat well.
Serve and enjoy.

Nutrition Info: Calories: 203 kcal Fat: 18 g Protein: 6 g Carbs: 6 g Fiber: 1 g

Greek pasta salad with cucumber and artichoke hearts

Preparation time: 5 minutes
Cooking time: 0 minute
Servings: 10

Ingredients:
½ cup olive oil
Four minced garlic cloves
1/4 cup white balsamic vinegar tbsp oregano
1 cup crumbled feta cheese
1 tsp ground pepper
15 oz sliced artichoke hearts
1 lb pasta noodles cooked
12 oz roasted and chopped red bell peppers
One sliced English cucumber
8 oz sliced Kalamata olives
¼ sliced red onion
1/3 cup chopped basil leaves
1 tsp kosher salt

Directions:
Combine vinegar, oregano, salt, olive oil, garlic, and black pepper in a bowl and mix well. Set aside.
In a big sized bowl, combine olives, onions, cheese, artichoke hearts, cooked pasta, cucumber and bell peppers,

Drizzle dressing over the artichoke hearts mixture and toss to coat. Garnish with feta cheese and basil and serve after half an hour.

Nutrition Info: Calories: 415.43 kcal Fat: 23.15 g Protein: 9.54 g Carbs: 42.54 g Fiber: 4.46 g

Quinoa and kale protein power salad

Preparation time: 5 minutes

Cooking time: 15 minutes

Servings: 5

Ingredients:

One sliced zucchini

½ tbsp extra virgin olive oil

¼ tsp turmeric

¼ tsp cumin

¼ tsp paprika tsp minced garlic,

One pinch of red pepper flakes

½ cup cooked quinoa

Salt to taste

1 cup drained chickpeas

1 cup chopped curly kale

Directions:

In a bowl, whisk chili flakes, cumin, paprika, salt, olive oil, garlic, and turmeric. Keep it aside.

Toast quinoa for one minute in olive oil.

Cook toasted quinoa following the instructions given over the package. Set aside.

Sauté garlic, kale, chickpeas, and zucchini in heated olive oil in the same skillet used to toast quinoa.

Cook for a few minutes until the mixture starts to sweat.

Sprinkle salt and remove skillet from flame.

In a bowl, combine veggies mixture and quinoa and leave for 10 minutes.

In a skillet, sauté spices in oil for two minutes and add in veggies mixture.

Serve and enjoy.

Nutrition Info: Calories: 106 kcal Fat: 3 g Protein: 5 g Carbs: 16 g Fiber: 4 g

Whole wheat Greek pasta salad

Preparation time: 15 minutes
Cooking time: 0 minute
Servings: 6

Ingredients:
1 lb rotini pasta
One chopped cucumber
1 cup sliced cherry tomatoes
One chopped yellow capsicum
1 cup chopped Kalamata olives
One diced red onion 2 tbsp chopped dill
½ cup feta cheese
Salt to taste
Black pepper to taste
Dressing
2minced garlic cloves
¼ cup olive oil
3tbsp red wine vinegar
½ lemon juice
Salt to taste
½ tsp oregano
Black pepper to taste

Directions:

Bring water to boil in a pot. Stir in salt and cook pasta in it until it is done.

Strain pasta and set aside.

Mix Olive oil, vinegar, salt, lemon juice, oregano, pepper, and garlic in a bowl. The dressing is ready.

Combine cooked pasta, cucumber, olives, feta cheese, onions, bell pepper, tomatoes, and dill in a salad serving bowl.

Drizzle dressing over the mixture and toss to coat.

Serve and enjoy it.

Nutrition Info: Calories: 437 kcal Fat: 16 g Protein: 14 g Carbs: 64 g Fiber: 2 g

Tomato and hearts of palm salad

Preparation time: 15 minutes
Cooking time: 0 minute
Servings: 4

Ingredients:
14 oz sliced hearts of palm, diced avocados tbsp lime juice cup sliced grape tomatoes
1/4 cup sliced green onion
1/2 cup chopped cilantro
Salt to taste

Directions:
In a bowl, combine drained and sliced palm hearts, lime juice, tomatoes, avocados, and onions.
Mix salt to adjust the taste.
Sprinkle cilantro to enhance the taste and serve.

Nutrition Info: Calories: 199 kcal Fat: 15 g Protein: 5 g Carbs: 15 g Fiber: 10 g

Quinoa tabbouleh with chickpeas

Preparation time: 20 minutes
Cooking time: 15 minutes
Servings: 8

Ingredients:

1 cup quinoa

2 cups of water

1.5 cups chickpeas cooked cups sliced cherry tomatoescups slicing cucumber

3/4 cups chopped parsley

2/3 cups chopped onions Tbsp chopped mint

Ground Pepper to taste

Dressing

1/3 cups olive oil lemon zest tbsp lemon juice

1.5 tsp minced garlic

¾ tsp salt

Directions:

In a bowl, mix lemon juice, salt, oil, lemon zest, and garlic. The dressing is ready.

In a deep pot, add two cups of water, a pinch of salt, and quinoa. Let it boil.

When the water starts boiling, lower the flame to low and cover. Let it simmer for about 15 minutes.

Strain quinoa and set aside to cool down.

In a bowl, combine onions, cucumbers, mint, tomatoes, cooked quinoa, parsley, black pepper, and chickpeas.

Add dressing in quinoa mixture and mix well.

Adjust flavor using black pepper and salt and serve.

Nutrition Info: : Calories: 206 kcal Fat: 12 g Protein: 5 g Carbs: 22 g Fiber: 3 g

Autumn couscous salad

Preparation time: 10 minutes
Cooking time: 25 minutes
Servings: 8

Ingredients:
Salad
1.5 cups dry pearl couscous
2 lb cubed butternut squash
1/2 cup dried cranberries
1/2 chopped red onion
sliced fennel bulb
tbsp olive oil bunch sliced kale
1/2 cup chopped pecans
Dressing
2 tbsp apple cider vinegar
1/3 cup olive oil
2 tbsp honey tbsp Dijon mustard
1 tbsp lemon juice
Kosher salt to taste tbsp orange juice
Black pepper to taste

Directions:
Put fennel, onions, and butternut squash over a baking tray lined with a parchment sheet.
Sprinkle salt, olive oil, and black pepper over butternut squash.

Bake in a preheated oven at 400 degrees for 30 minutes.
Cook couscous by following the instructions given on the package.

Mix mustard, olive oil, juice, vinegar, honey, salt, and black pepper in a jar and shake until the mixture emulsifies. The dressing is ready.

In a bowl, combine baked veggies, kale, pecans, couscous, and cranberries. Pour dressing over the mixture and toss well. Serve and enjoy it.

Nutrition Info: Calories: 266 kcal Fat: 21 g Protein: 4 g Carbs: 18 g Fiber: 3 g

Slow cooker chicken cacciatore

Preparation time: 15 minutes
Cooking time: 240 minutes
Servings: 5

Ingredients:
Three chopped garlic cloves
1.5 tbsp olive oil
1.25 tbsp balsamic vinegar
1 tsp kosher salt
1/2 tsp black pepper
2 tsp Italian seasoning
28 oz crushed tomatoes
2 lb boneless chicken breastschopped yellow onion
One chopped green bell pepper
8 oz sliced cremini mushrooms

Directions:
Rub the chicken with salt and black pepper and cook in heated oil in a skillet over a high flame for five minutes from both sides. Shift the chicken to the slow cooker.
Sauté onions in heated oil for three minutes in a skillet over medium flame.
Stir in vinegar and garlic and cook for one more minute.
Shift the garlic mixture to the slow cooker.

Add mushrooms, tomatoes, Italian seasoning, and bell pepper and mix.

Cover the cooker and cook on low flame for four hours.

After chicken is done, sprinkle salt, vinegar, and pepper and serve with rice or whatever you like.

Nutrition Info: Calories: 228 kcal Fat: 8 g Protein: 32 g Carbs: 10 g Fiber: 3 g

Greek baked cod with lemon and garlic

Preparation time: 10 minutes
Cooking time: 12 minutes
Servings: 4

Ingredients:

Five minced garlic cloves 1.5 lb Cod fillet

¼ cup chopped parsley

Lemon Juice Mixture

5 tbsp Olive oil

5 tbsp lemon juice

2 tbsp butter

Coating

1/3 cup all-purpose flour

¾ tsp salt

¾ tsp paprika 1 tsp coriander

¾ tsp cumin

½ tsp black pepper

Directions:

In a medium-sized bowl, combine olive oil, butter, and lemon juice and keep it aside. Whisk flour, salt, spices, and pepper in a bowl and keep it aside.

Coat fish with lemon mixture followed by coating with flour mixture.

Sauté coated fish in heated olive oil in a skillet over medium flame for two minutes from each side. Mix garlic into lemon juice and pour over sautéed fish.

Bake in a preheated oven at 400 degrees for almost 10 minutes. Drizzle parsley and serve with your favorite salad or rice.

Nutrition Info: Calories: 312 kcal Fat: 18.4 g Protein: 23.1 g Carbs: 16.1 g Fiber: 14 g

Moroccan fish

Preparation time: 10 minutes
Cooking time: 30 minutes
Servings: 6

Ingredients:
Olive oil as required
2 tbsp tomato paste
Eight minced garlic cloves
Two diced tomatoes
½ tsp cumin
15 oz chickpeas sliced red pepper cup water
Kosher salt to taste
Handful of cilantros
Black pepper to taste
1.5 lb cod fillet pieces
1.5 tsp allspice mixture
¾ tsp paprika
1 tbsp lemon juice
½ sliced lemon

Directions:
Sauté garlic in heated oil for one minute.
Stir in bell pepper and diced tomatoes and tomato paste and cook for five minutes over medium flame with constant stirring.

Mix garlic, salt, chickpeas, cilantro, pepper, water, and half tsp of allspice mixture. Let it boil and reduce the flame and simmer for 20 minutes.

Whisk leftover allspice mixture, paprika, salt, cumin, and pepper in a bowl.

Rub fish with spice mixture and oil.

Place fish and fish mixture in a pan, followed by a cooked chickpea mixture, lemon slices, and juice.

Let it cook for 15 minutes over low flame.

Sprinkle cilantro and serve.

Sprinkle spice mixture over the fish

Nutrition Info: Calories: 463 kcal Fat: 5.7 g Protein: 23.7 g Carbs: 67.2 g Fiber: 2.3 g

Lemon garlic salmon

Preparation time: 10 minutes
Cooking time: 18 minutes
Servings: 6

Ingredients:
Salmon
2 lb salmon fillet
2 tbsp parsley for garnishing
Olive oil
Kosher salt
½ sliced lemon
Lemon-Garlic Sauce
Zest of one lemon
3 tbsp olive oil
3 tbsp of lemon juice
Five chopped garlic cloves tsp sweet paprika tsp dry oregano
½ tsp black pepper

Directions:
In a bowl, whisk olive oil, pepper, garlic, lemon zest and juice, oregano, and paprika in a mixing bowl and set aside. The lemon garlic sauce is ready.
Brush baking tray with oil lined with foil paper.
Place seasoned (with salt) salmon on a baking tray and pour the sauce over the salmon.

Bake in a preheated oven at 375 degrees for 20 minutes.

Broil baked salmon for three minutes and serve after garnishing.

Nutrition Info: Calories: 338 kcal Fat: 25.8 g Protein: 33.1 g Carbs: 11.8 g Fiber: 3 g

Sheet pan chicken and vegetables

Preparation time: 15 minutes
Cooking time: 45 minutes
Servings: 6

Ingredients:

2 lb red potatoes

2 tbsp olive oil

One chopped onion

Three minced garlic cloves

1 tsp powdered rosemary

1.25 tsp salt

3/4 tsp pepper

Six chicken thighs

1/2 tsp paprika

6 cups baby spinach

Directions:

Mix onion, rosemary, potatoes, oil, salt, garlic, and pepper in a bowl.
Shift the potato mixture into a baking tray sprayed with oil.
Combine salt, pepper, paprika, and rosemary in another bowl and sprinkle over chicken.
Place chicken pieces over potato mixture and bake in a preheated oven at 425 degrees for 35 minutes.
Take chicken out of oven and place in serving dish.

Put spinach over veggies and bake for another ten minutes. Transfer cooked veggies over chicken and serve.

Nutrition Info: Calories: 357 kcal Fat: 14 g Protein: 28 g Carbs: 28 g Fiber: 4 g

www.ingramcontent.com/pod-product-compliance
Lightning Source LLC
Chambersburg PA
CBHW070729030426
42336CB00013B/1928